Herbal Healing

Remedies for Your Most Common Illnesses

Disclaimer

How This Book is Helpful for You!

Medicines and allopathic treatments seem to be getting more expensive each day. This is the reason why more and more people are turning to home remedies for common diseases and ailments. The purpose of writing this book is just that, to allow you to cure common illnesses right at home, without having to rush to the doctor's office every time you sneeze or your toddler hiccups.

This nook will inform you about the following things:

1. What herbal remedies are, how they work and why they are better than any other kind of treatment.
2. Step by step recipes for treating a variety of common diseases, ailments and medical conditions.
3. All the ingredients are easily available in your kitchen or garden.
4. Some additional information about how you can improvise in a situation where you might not have some particular ingredient at hand.

By the time you are done reading this book, you will no longer have to worry about the change in weather or the cuts and scrapes your child gets when they play hard. It is of course advised that you be careful about using products that you might be allergic to. Also make sure you test the remedy before ingesting or putting it on.

So let us dive into the healthy, side-effect less and inexpensive world of herbal remedies.

Contents

Introduction

Most people don't think that herbal remedies can actually work. And this is where they are entirely wrong. It's true that herbal remedies give results that are slower than allopathic medication, but the effects of herbal healing are more long lasting and have absolutely no side effects. Perhaps the best thing about them is the fact that they can easily be prepared at home and you don't have to spend hundreds or thousands of dollars, yet get little or no benefit at all.

The interesting part to note is that even though people generally tend to disregard the advantages of herbal remedies, approximately 80% of the population uses herbal healing for some cause or the other. Some of the herbs that are most popularly used include saw palmetto, aloe, garlic, goldenseal, Echinacea, ginseng, ginkgo, ephedra, and cranberry. These herbs help in improving a variety of conditions.

So if you are not a believer in the power of herbal healing, do not underestimate its effects. From headaches, to colds, flu to rashes, allergies to bruises, herbal remedies can work better than even the medicines a doctor gives you. Below we have compiled a list of recipes that can easily be prepared at home and used without the added worries of coming to any kind of harm.

Here are all the herbal remedies for you and your family to feel at ease.

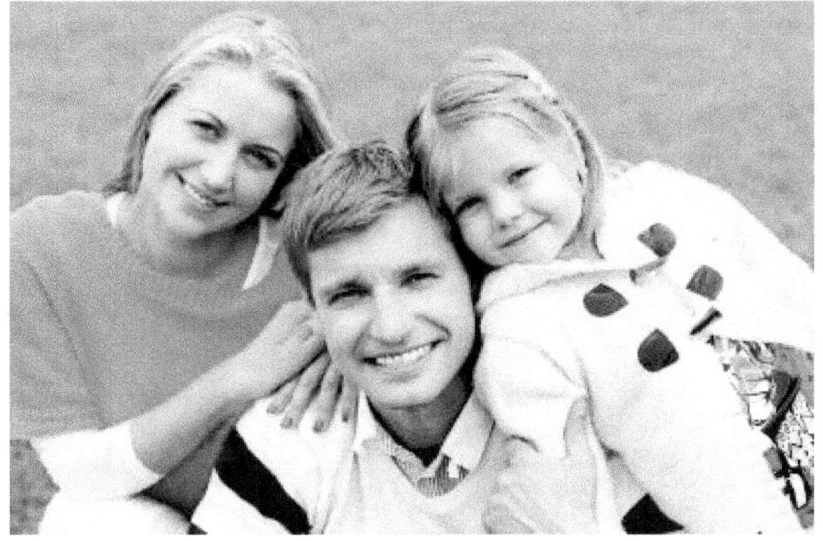

Flu and Cold

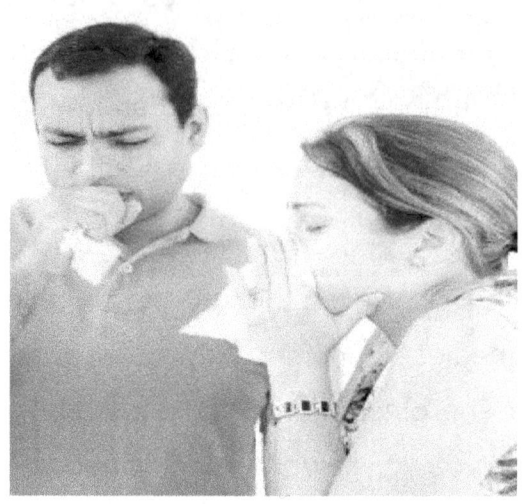

Flu and cold are some of the most commonly occurring problems all over the world. From children to adults, toddlers to seniors, it can be a nuisance for everyone. Research suggests that medication may stop the condition for a while, but ultimately they are not beneficial as a cure. It can also be rightly said that it is better to treat colds and flu with herbal medicine because their effect would be harmless. Here are some easy recipes to cure flu and cold.

1. Lemony Spray

Try making and using this lemon spray to help soothe your itching throat and torturing flu.

Ingredients

¼ cup of lemon juice

15 drops of lemon essential oil

3 drops of peppermint essential oil

¼ cup water

Methods

Simply combine all the ingredients together and store in a small spray bottle. All you will have to do is spray some in your throat and store it in the fridge so that it can last long. Don't use the mixture for more than 2 weeks.

2. Mixed Herb Tea

There are plenty of herbs that you can use to make yourself a warm concoction to ease the flu as well as cold symptoms. This one is better because it will also help lower the fever and congestion in your chest. The ingredients are easily available at health food stores and organic stores.

Ingredients

½ teaspoon of Schisandra berries

½ teaspoon of Echinacea root

½ teaspoon of elder flowers

½ teaspoon of yarrow flowers

½ teaspoon of peppermint leaves

3 cups of boiling water

Methods

Mix all the ingredients together and boil them. Strain the liquid and drink it up. All you will have to do is drink the tea at least 2 - 3 times a day and feel engulfed in warm comfort.

3. Tincture a la Echinacea

This is just the herb to use if you have been suffering from flu and cold for long. It is best that you start using the tincture as soon as you feel that you are about to come down with the condition. Echinacea is easily available in pill form, but it is better that you use it in the form of this tincture.

Ingredients

A quart jar

Echinacea blossoms, enough to fill 2/3 of the jar

80-proof apple cider vinegar or vodka solution

Methods

Take the quart jar and put blossoms in it. Then pour vodka or vinegar on top, so that all the flowers are soaked. Cover tightly and store in a cool and dark place for 2 weeks or so. After 2 weeks, strain the liquid and store in the fridge. Whenever there is need, all you have to do is mix a teaspoon of the tincture into your drink, be it tea, juice or water and drink it three times a day. You will notice your flu getting better in a day.

4. Vapor Rub

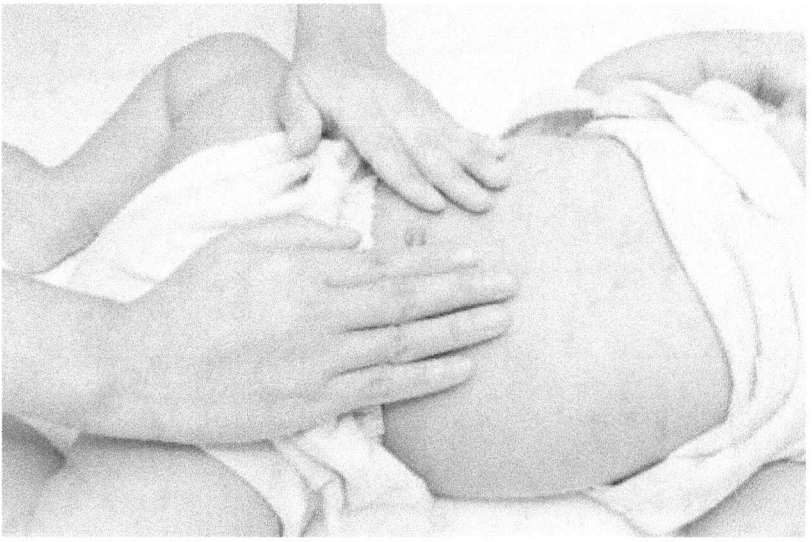

Vapor rubs are great for kids, as well as adults. They work wonderfully for sore throats, flu and colds. Imagine how much better the vapor-rub would be, if you make it yourself with herbal ingredients. Here is an easy recipe for you.

Ingredients

1/8 cup of olive oil

10 drops of peppermint essential oil

3 drops of thyme essential oil

10 drops of eucalyptus essential oil

Methods

Mix all of the oils well and rub it on chest, temples and throat. Cover to keep the areas warm. The vapor rub will help you sleep easily and clear the congestion in your throat.

5. Bee Pollen

Bee pollen is also believed to be the perfect cure for not only flu and cold but also helps your immune system into becoming stronger. You will notice that when you start using bee pollen, the chances of acquiring infections and other autoimmune disease decreases significantly. But those aren't the only ailments that bee pollen is great for. It helps to stave off cancer, lower blood pressure and help fight off skin problems.

Ingredients

½ a teaspoon of bee pollen

Glass of milk

Methods

All you will need to do is mix the pollen in milk, warm it up and drink it. You can even add the pollen in your regular cereal or oatmeal breakfast.

6. Herb Steam Inhalation

Steam can sometimes work better than any other medicine, especially if you are among those people who have sinusitis or congestion. Taking steam with plain water makes you feel better for a while, but if you add an assortment of herbs to it, the relief you get is long lasting. Here is how you can make an herbal inhalation.

Ingredients

A length of cheesecloth or some other soft material

1 teaspoon of chamomile

1 teaspoon of thyme

1 teaspoon of eucalyptus

Very hot water in a large bowl or sink

Methods

You can either take the water in a large bowl or pour it in your sink. Put all the herbs in the cloth and tie them in a way that it starts resembling a tea bag. Put it in the hot water and stir the water a little. Lean into the bowl or sink, keeping your face a safe distance from the water and cover your head with a towel. Take deep breaths. Repeat the process as necessary. The effects are instantaneous. You will feel your sinus clearing and even your headache will disappear.

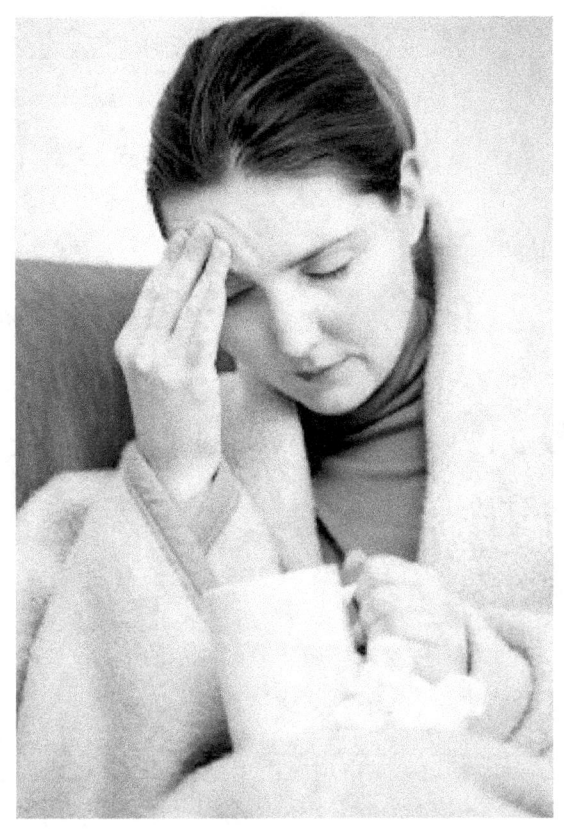

Acid Reflux and Heart Burn

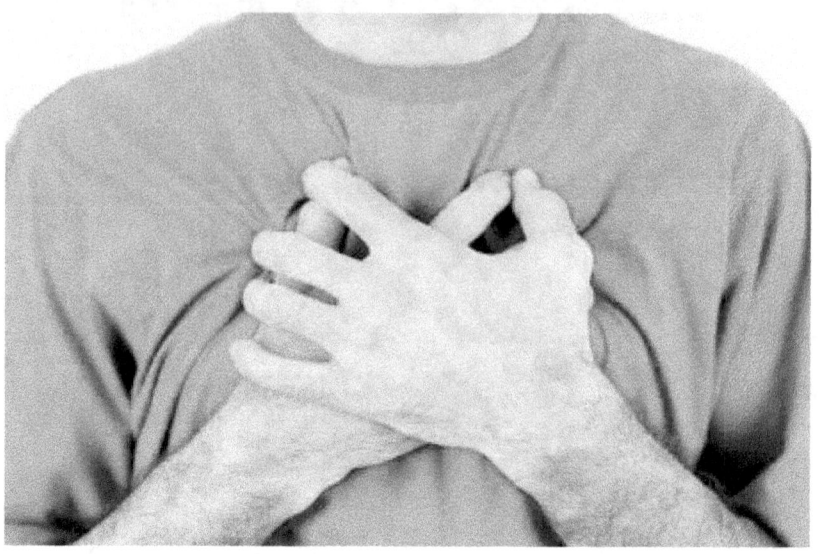

1. <u>Baking Soda & Turmeric Reliever</u>

You must have heard the old wives tale that states that baking soda is the best way to beat heartburn. Add a little turmeric to the mixture and you are good to go. But research suggests that taking baking soda once in a while is ok, too much of it can be harmful and cause nausea.

Ingredients

½ teaspoon of baking soda

¼ teaspoon of turmeric

½ glass of water at room temperature

Methods

Mix the herbs in water and drink it up. Within half an hour your acidity and heart burn will dissolve. The reason why this works is because baking soda is a bicarbonate which is alkaline in nature and neutralizes the effect of acid in your stomach.

2. Heart-Burn Easing Tea

Tea may not seem like the best thing to ingest when you feel like throwing up, but this one can help with the acidity and nausea. It is very easy to make and if you don't have one ingredient you can either leave it or replace it by something else.

Ingredients

1 teaspoon of freshly grated ginger root

1 teaspoon of fennel seeds

A pinch of cinnamon

1 cup water

Methods

Boil the water and add all the herbs to it. Let steep for 10 minutes, drain and drink it up. Not only will the heartburn ease, you will also feel lighter and the nausea will stop completely. You can eliminate any of the herbs that do not suit you or is not at home and replace it with anise, caraway or cardamom.

3. Marshmallow Root Concoction

Marshmallow root is considered to be one of the most effective remedies for acid reflux and heartburn. You can also add some other ingredients to make it even more functional. Here is an easy way to make the drink.

Ingredients

2 teaspoons of marshmallow root

1 teaspoon of chamomile

1 teaspoon of catnip

1 teaspoon of plantain leaf

1 teaspoon of fennel

2 glasses of water

Methods

Heat up the water and add all the herbs to it. Mix and let sit for 10 minutes. Strain and use. You can either drink the concoction warm as a type of tea or refrigerate it and drink it cold. Make sure you drink it twice in one day.

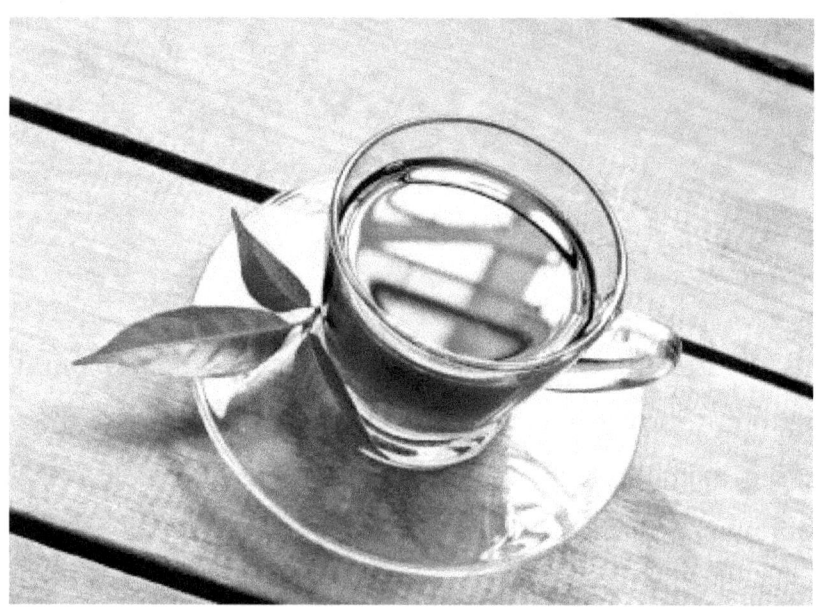

Headaches

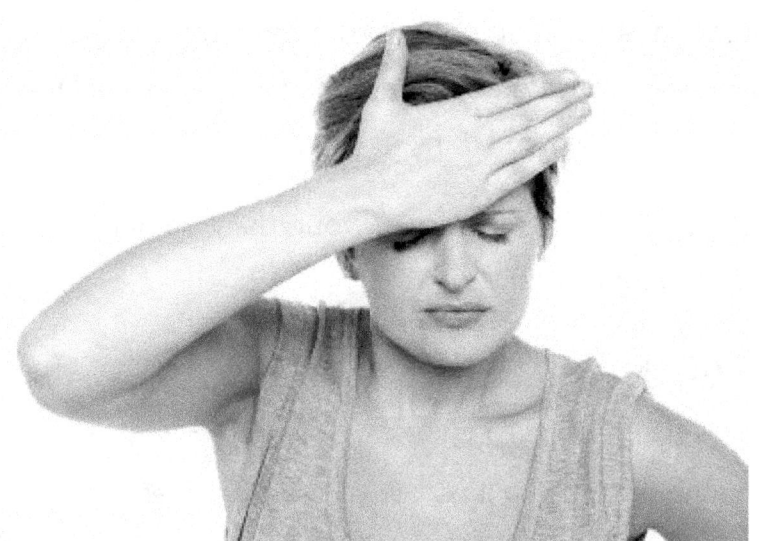

1. <u>Migraine Relieving Tea</u>

Headaches are bad but migraines can become the doom of your existence. The worst thing about migraine is that there is no cure. You can take medicines and they may or may not provide temporary relief, but they are always looming over your head. This is the reason that using herbal treatments is better than opting for medication. This herbal tea is bound to reduce stress and the awful pain.

Ingredients

4 teaspoons chamomile flowers

1 teaspoon passion flowers

2 teaspoons feverfew

1 teaspoon skullcap

1 teaspoon lemon balm

¼ ginger root

Water

Methods

Mix all of the herbs together thoroughly and store in an airtight jar. Whenever you have the migraine, take one cup water, boil it and add 1 teaspoon of the herb mixture in it. Let steep for 8-10 minutes, strain and drink.

If you start drinking this tea as part of your daily routine, you will notice a visible difference in your migraine condition.

2. Butter-Minty Massage Oil

Sounds yummy, doesn't it? It actually works wonders too. It is easy to make and you can store it for a long time, using it as per your requirements.

Ingredients

10 drops of peppermint essential oil

5 drops of willow extract

5 drops of butterbur root extract

5 tablespoons of a base oil, coconut, olive or almond

Methods

Combine all the oils well and store in a glass bottle. Whenever you feel a headache coming on, rub the oil on temples, forehead and massage some in your hair too. But massage the oil in hair very lightly. Leave on for some time and when the pain is gone, you can wash it off with warm water.

3. Cayenne Rosemary Balm

Cayenne pepper is believed to be a cure for not only headaches and migraines, but also shoulder and neck aches. Keep in mind though that you are not supposed to ingest it, rather just apply to the place where the pain is.

Ingredients

½ teaspoon of cayenne powder

A few drops of rosemary essential oil

A few drops of juniper oil

3 tablespoons of olive or almond oil

Methods

Mix all of the ingredients thoroughly and store in an airtight bottle. Whenever you experience a headache massage this balm on the nape of your neck, shoulders and upper back. Keep on massaging until all the muscles have gotten relaxed. Just make sure that you are not allergic to any of the ingredients by first checking on a small patch of skin.

4. Stimulating Tea

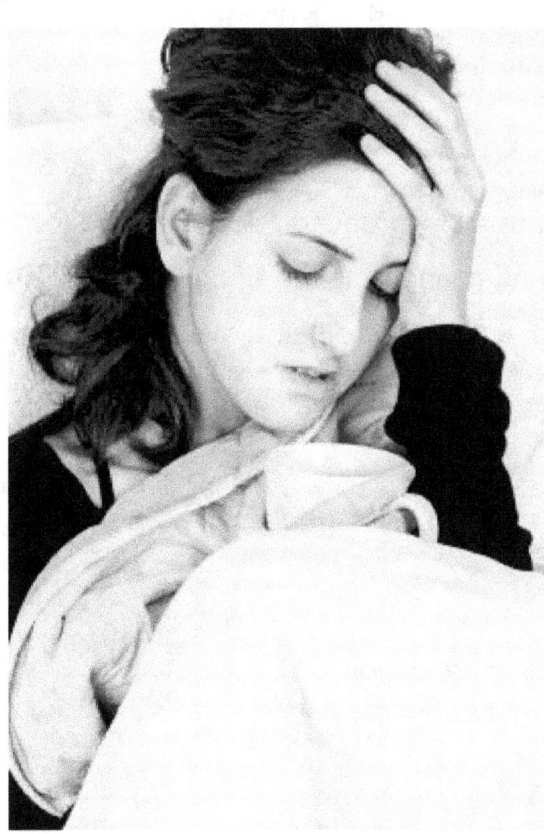

Ingredients

20 grams of fresh ginger

40 grams of fresh Herba Mentha or peppermint

10 grams of brown sugar or honey

Peppermint, as per taste

½ liters of water

Methods

Mix together sugar/ honey and ginger. Add water and bring the mixture to a boil. Once it starts boiling, lower the heat and let simmer for about 30 minutes. Add in peppermint and cook for another 5 minutes. Strain and drink while hot. You can drink as much as you like. It will not only relieve the headache but will also stimulate your nerves, making you feel fresh and energetic.

5. Clovy Cinnamon Relief

Cloves and cinnamons are both great for headaches. They work by neutralizing the effects of the headache and giving a sense of lightness. Try it and see the effects. Just don't use the oil if you are sensitive to either cloves or cinnamon.

Ingredients

10 ml of cinnamon oil

3 grams of crushed cloves

A few drops of peppermint essential oil

Methods

Combine all of the ingredients and then apply to forehead and temples. Massage gently and then lie down for a while. You will notice that within 10 minutes the pain starts dissipating.

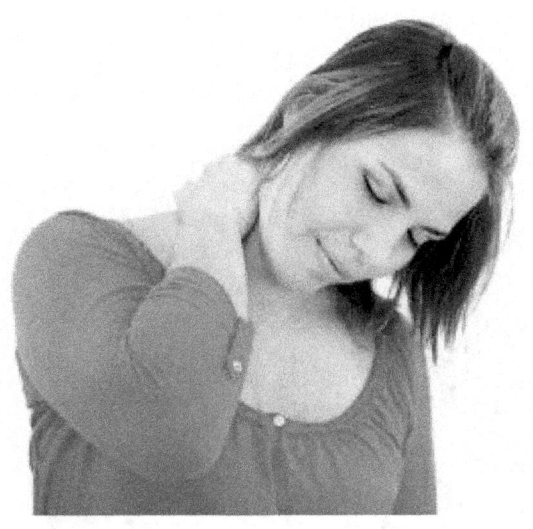

Diarrhea

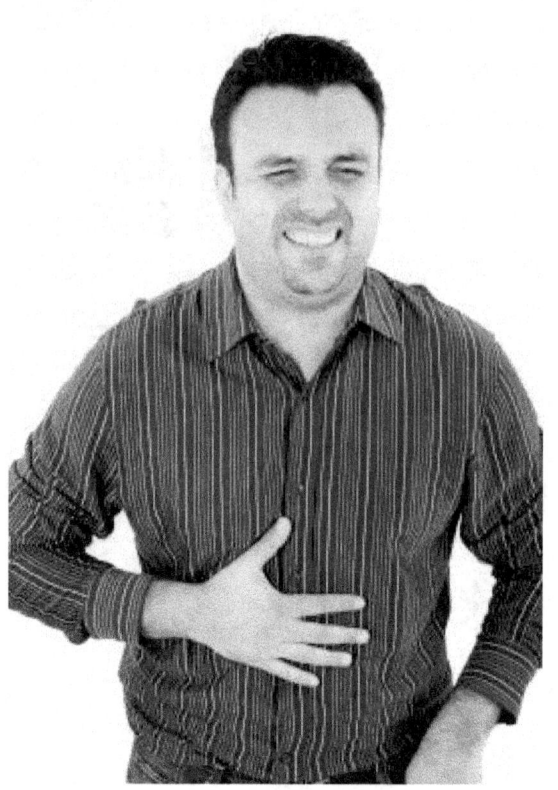

1. <u>Chamomile Tea</u>

Diarrhea can become very painful if not treated in time. The painkillers or antibiotics that are prescribed by the doctor may be useful, but they can cause harmful side effects. If your condition is not too adverse, it is better that you handle the problem with herbal healing. Chamomile tea is great because it reduces the intestinal inflammation. Here is how you can make it.

Ingredients

1 teaspoon chamomile flowers

1 teaspoon peppermint leaves

1 teaspoon of dried blackberry leaves

Methods

Take 1 1/2 cups of water and bring it to a boil. Add all the herbs to it and let steep for 10 minutes. Strain and drink this tea and you will notice a difference almost immediately. You can consume this tea twice a day.

2. Fenugreek Tonic

This remedy should never be tried with kids as their stomachs are too sensitive. Therefore, if your toddler has diarrhea, don't give this tonic to them. But it can work wonderfully for adults. Just try half a cup first and if it works, you can take two cups of this tonic a day.

Ingredients

½ teaspoon of fenugreek seeds

½ teaspoon of nettles

½ teaspoon of fennel

Water

Methods

Heat up water with fennel and when it starts boiling, switch off the heat. Add other herbs to it and let sit for 15 minutes. Strain and drink up. You can make this tonic in greater quantity, store it in the fridge and drink it throughout the day. Don't consume more than 2 glasses per day.

3. Honeydote

Honey is not just great for your sore throat, but also works for a sore or sour stomach. The best part? Diarrhea stops.

Ingredients

1 tablespoon of honey

A pinch of cinnamon powder

½ teaspoon of ginger powder

½ teaspoon of cumin powder

½ teaspoon of cinnamon powder

Methods

Mix all the herbs & honey and take the tonic three times a day. The first day will show results!

4. Pomegranate Rice

Rice is made of starch, which is what makes it great. It covers the lining of the stomach making it stronger and resistant to infections and bacteria. Try this recipe to achieve great results.

Ingredients

½ cup of white rice

½ teaspoon of ginger paste

½ cup of pomegranate juice

4 cups of water

Salt as per taste

Methods

Make the rice with water, salt and ginger paste. Once done, add the pomegranate juice and eat as much as you want. Not only is this gruel tasty, it also controls the bowel movement and reduces inflammation of the intestine walls. Another great thing is that it restores energy to the body.

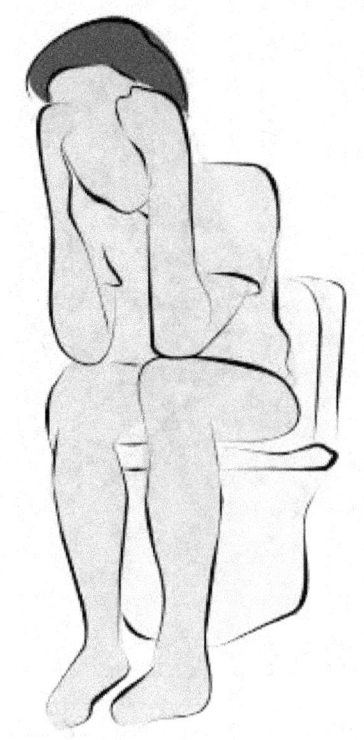

Aches and Pains

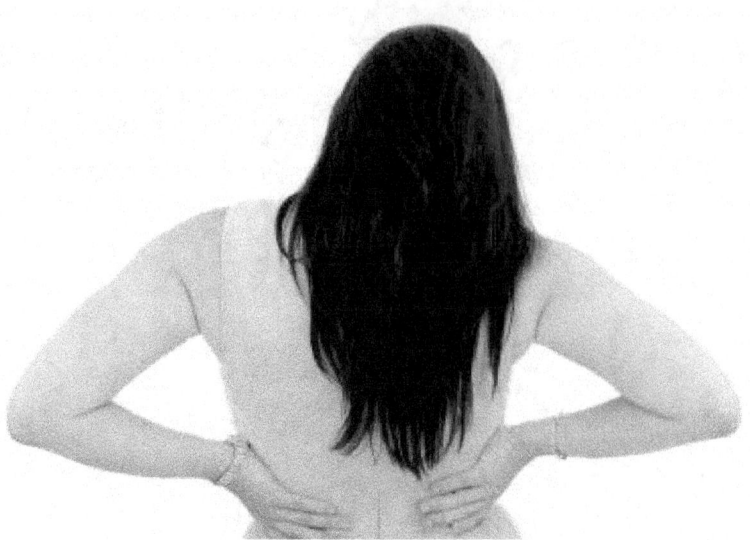

1. <u>Eucalyptus Muscle Massage Oil</u>

Muscle pain can become truly painful if it continues to take place. Instead of letting things get worse, here is how you can handle the pain.

Ingredients

15 ml of your choice of a carrier oil, olive, almond or coconut

5 drops of Bay laurel essential oil

3 drops of Ylang Ylang essential oil

4 drops of Rosemary essential oil

Methods

Mix all of the oils well and store in a glass jar. Rub with soft hands on the muscles for as long as it takes to relax them. Leave on and try to keep the muscles warm. Whenever the pain gets bad, you can have a rub of this wonder oil.

2. Fatigue Relieving Grapefruit Goodness

Grapefruit may be a miracle cure for obesity, but it works on many other levels. When it comes to fatigue, whether you eat it or put it on, it will help you shed the stress and feel rejuvenated all over again.

Ingredients

20 ml of carrier oil, your choice

5 drops of Palmarosa essential oil

8 drops of Grapefruit essential oil

3 drops of Thyme essential oil

Methods

Mix all of the oils well and apply to whichever area is aching. Do not rub hard, just massage with a soft hand. You will notice a visible difference within no time!

3. Minty Refreshment

Mint is not only great for your throat and head; it also works wonders for the overall well being of the body. This massage oil will help ease the ache in your body and leave you feeling refreshed.

Ingredients

20 ml of carrier oil, preferably almond or olive oil

3 drops of lavender essential oil

6 drops of peppermint essential oil

3 drops of Bergamot

3 drops of lemon juice

A pinch of basil

Methods

Combine all of the ingredients together and leave the mixture overnight. The oil will get infused properly. Then whenever you feel too stressed out and have aches in various body parts, massage this oil and see the effects. The combination of mint and lemon will help you feel relaxed and refreshed.

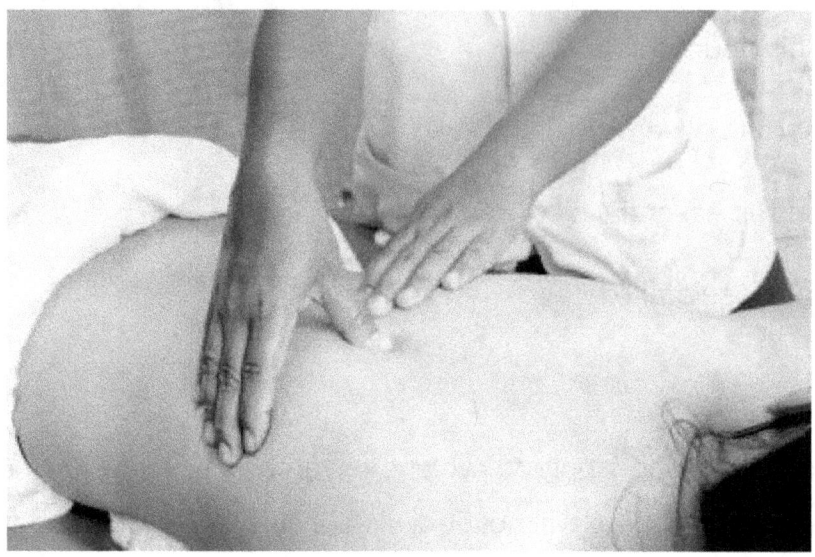

Allergies Solution

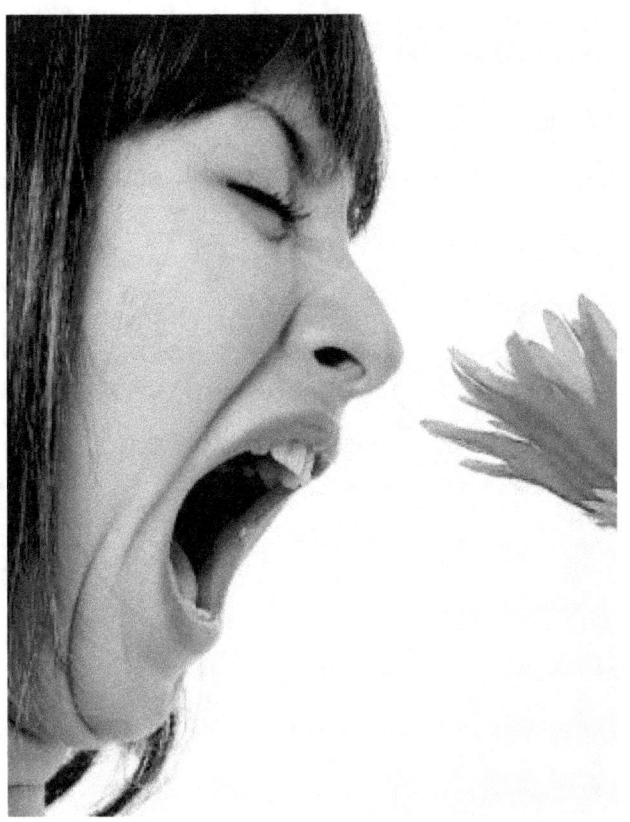

1. Seasonal Allergies Tincture

Whenever the weather changes, people who suffer from allergies feel like living in a bubble. The runny nose, the constant sneezing and in some extreme cases, rashes are very inconvenient. This tincture will help you with all kinds of seasonal allergies and you will not have to get closeted in your house.

Ingredients

1 part of Oregon grape

2 parts of Ambrosia

2 parts of Horehound

3 parts of Bayberry

4 parts of Yerba Masa

4 parts of Yerba Santa

Methods

You have the choice of either mixing the herbs as tinctures or tincture it at 1:5, 60% alcohol. Whenever there is a change in the season, start using 30-60 drops 2 times a day.

2. <u>De Congest Your Chest</u>

People who suffer from allergies do not only have a runny nose, but severe cases also give birth to coughs and cold. This tea is great for a runny nose, a congested chest or cough and cold. Try taking it to see the results.

Ingredients

2 parts of cubeb berries

3 parts of Ma Huang

3 parts of coltsfoot leaves

3 parts of Mormon Tea

3 parts of Yerba Santa

Methods

Mix all of the herbs in water and bring to a boil. Let cool slightly, drink it up. There may be times when the tea infusion makes you feel too sleepy or anxious. If that happens try taking Ma Huang out.

3. <u>Allergy Ridding Soup</u>

Allergies can be a real downer. If you have been feeling down and don't know how to step out of the house, try using this soup. Not only will it ease the allergies, it will also make you energetic and calm.

Ingredients

1 small onion

1 clove of garlic

1 ½ cup of leaves and taproot of evening primrose

1 cup of nettle leaves

1 cup of celery stalks

Vinegar, salt, black pepper, turmeric, curry powder and celery seeds to taste

Methods

Boil the onion and garlic with their peelings. Then add the evening primrose to it and let it cook for a while, about 5 minutes. Then add nettles and diced celery stalks for 5-10 minutes on low heat. Your soup is ready. Remove the onion skin and garlic peel. Season with the rest of the ingredients and consume immediately. You will notice a sense of uplifting comes over you. Drink it as many days as you like.

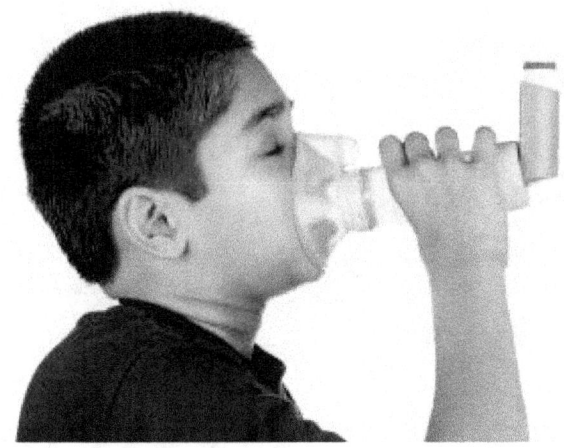

Nerves, Anxiety and Depression

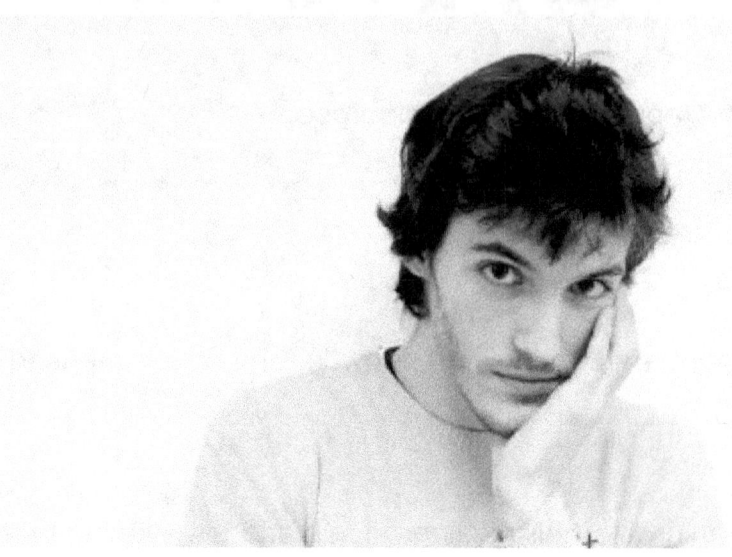

1. <u>Serenity Tea</u>

There are many times that you feel extremely anxious and don't know how to get rid of the nerves. Be it the upcoming state exams or the marriage of your daughter, simple job test anxiety or fear of the unknown, this tea will help you in all situations. It is recommended that you not drink it if you are pregnant or do not want to fall asleep.

Ingredients

3 parts of catnip

3 parts of chamomile flowers

3 parts of passion flower

2 parts of spearmint

2 parts of hops

2 parts of lemon balm

1 part of viscum album

Methods

Combine all of the ingredients in water and boil. It works best in evenings and right before going to sleep. You will notice that the anxiety gets alleviated immediately.

2. Jump Nerves Tonic

Have you been feeling jumpy? Is it because of the exam you are going to sit out the rest of the day? Feeling the stress palpitations coming on because of having to walk up to the alter and say 'I do'? Well this tonic can really do wonders for you.

Ingredients

½ ounce of fresh Selenicereus

5 ounces of passiflora FE

1 ounce of crataegus

1 ounce of verbena hastate

1 ounce of Hypericum

1 ounce of Leonurus cardiaca

Methods

Make the tonic from separate tinctures and use no more than 60-90 drops per dose. The tonic is not just excellent for the nerves but also for physical jumping sensation.

3. Un Depress Yourself

Depression can become a real problem if not handled in the right way, at the right time. Therefore, if you feel the first signs of depression, try this tincture and see it working out for you. You will notice a difference almost immediately. Make sure you keep on it until you feel completely better again.

Ingredients

1 part of Panaz quinquefolim

4 parts of Licorice Root

6 parts of fresh hypericum

2 parts of fresh oplopanax

5 parts of fresh Aralia berries

Methods

Mix all of the ingredients as tinctures. Use 60-90 drops for 3 times each day. It works great for depression with dry mucosa.

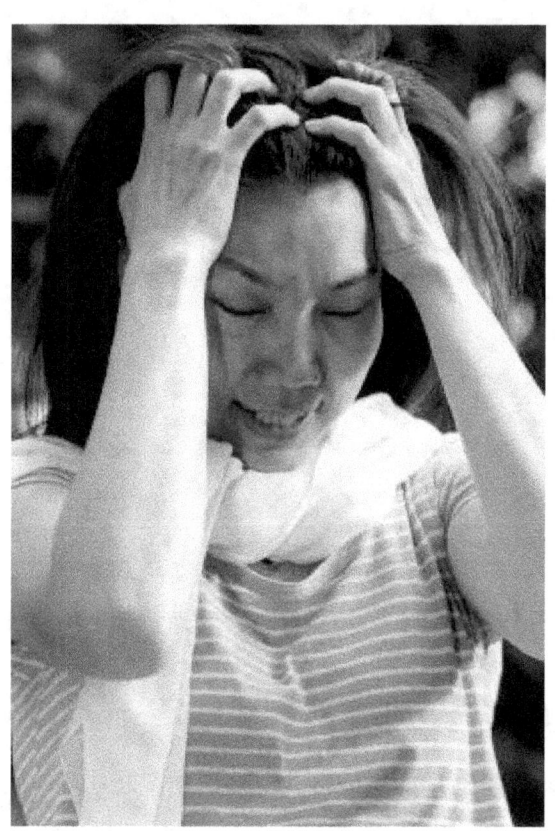

Cuts, Bruises and Stings

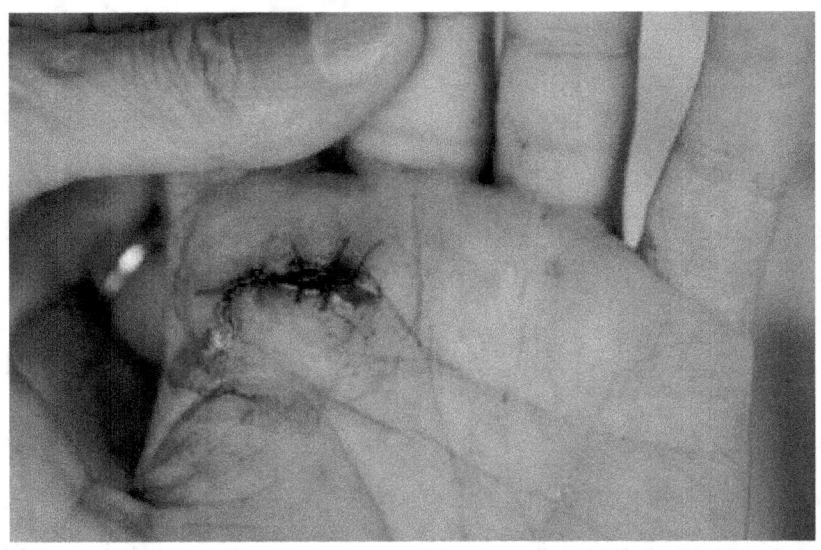

1. <u>A Salve to Heal</u>

If you have kids in the house then you will know how many cuts, bruises, scrapes, bug bites, bee stings, dry patches, scratches and other such incidents occur in a household. Even if you don't have kids that are the type who keeps banging in all the wrong places, this healing salve can be the perfect thing to keep in your house. You can even present it as a gift that you made with your sweat and blood!

Ingredients

1 ½ ounces of olive oil that is infused with Calendula Flowers

1 ounce olive oil that is infused with Plantain

1 ounce olive oil that is infused with goldenseal

½ ounce beeswax

½ teaspoon of rosemary antioxidant

1 tablespoon of tamanu oil

15 drops of tea tree oil

15 drops of lavender essential oil

Methods

Mix together all of the oils, beeswax and tamanu oil in a cup. Give this cup a warm water bath on a stove until the beeswax melts completely. Once all is in liquid form, remove from heat and add in the rosemary, tea tree and lavender oils. Store in a tightly lidded jar. Let cool and use as per need.

2. Blister Solving Salve

This salve can work wonderfully for all kinds of sores, blisters, stings, vaginitis, anal fissures, swellings and hemorrhoids. Don't use the mixture if you are allergic to any of the ingredients and try on a small patch of skin before using on any sensitive parts.

Ingredients

3 ounces of alcohol

7 ounces of beeswax

35 ounces of olive oil

5 ounces of Echinacea purpurea flowerheads

Methods

Make sure you remove the roots of the Echinacea flowers. Put the flower in a stainless steel container; pour alcohol on top and cover. Let sit for about 3 hours. Then add in the olive oil and blend. You should blend at a speed that the side of the container gets warmed up. Filter this mixture through muslin. Then heat up the oil in a double boiler, add beeswax and let simmer until the wax melts completely. Store in a glass container.

3. Wart Ointment

This ointment works extraordinarily well for venereal warts and herpes sores. So if you just had them or someone you know had them, whip it up and make their day! You will notice the pain going away and the marks fading in a short time.

Ingredients

10 Rosin or Colophony

5 ounces of myrrh tincture

12 ounces of olive oil

8 ounces of podophyllum root

Some beeswax pellets

Methods

You will have to percolate the podophyllum root in 95% alcohol to attain a 1:2 tincture. Then add myrrh tincture to it and evaporate on low heat so that 2 fluid of it is left. Then include rosin and olive oil and allow dispersing. Check to see if it sets on a metal surface and then add 1 ounce of beeswax if need be. Pour into jars, let cool and use!

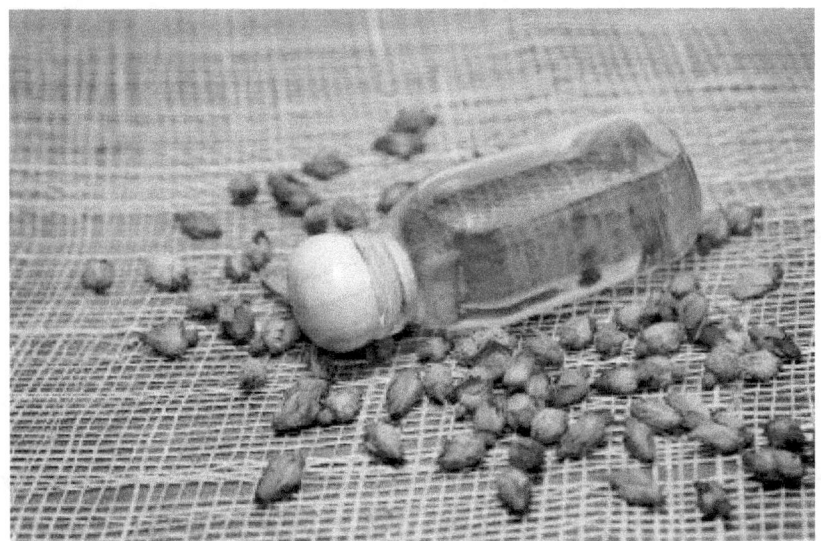

Eczema Problems

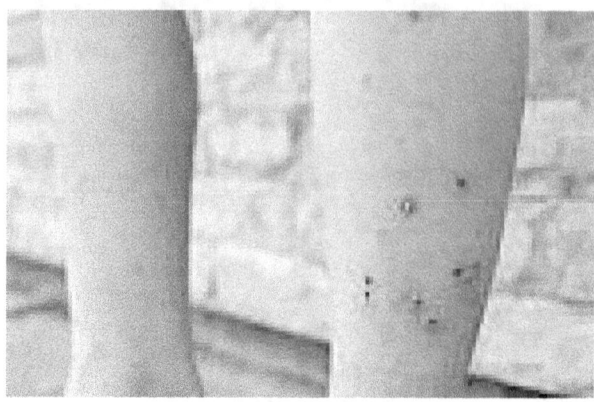

1. Eczema Solution

Eczema is not only painful, it also looks hideous. Also it can last a lifetime if not treated in time. Most medicines only reduce the condition but never seem to fully heal it. Try this herbal treatment and have results that are long lasting.

Ingredients

4 tablespoons of almond oil

½ teaspoon of turmeric

Few drops of geranium essential oil

Few drops of hyssop essential oil

Methods

Mix all of the ingredients together and apply wherever you have the eczema. Rub lightly and leave to dry. Keep applying twice every day for best results.

2. Tea Cure for Eczema

Applying something externally may not be the cure for your condition. Sometimes there are external factors that give cause for the eczema to flourish. If they are not treated properly, then eczema would keep returning every time. Drink this tea and see the effects. This tea is particularly great for scaling skin. The best part is that it can be consumed and applied to the affected area.

Ingredients

A handful of burdock leaves

Some yellow dock

A few heartsease (viola)

Some red clovers

Methods

Boil water and put the herbs in it. Let steep for 10 minutes and then drink the tea three times a day. You can also apply this tea on the eczema for greater results.

3. Dandelion Mixture

This mixture is great not just for eczema but many other skin conditions. It contains herbs that increase the elasticity and suppleness of the skin, removing inflammation, redness and soreness.

Ingredients

2 teaspoons of aloe vera gel (fresh)

1 teaspoon of dandelion milk

A few crushed horsetails

A few crushed milk thistles

Methods

Mix all of the ingredients well and apply to the affected areas. You will notice that within a day or two the redness has decreased and skin seems to be less irritated. Make sure you try the mixture on a small skin patch to know that it does not cause any reaction to your skin.

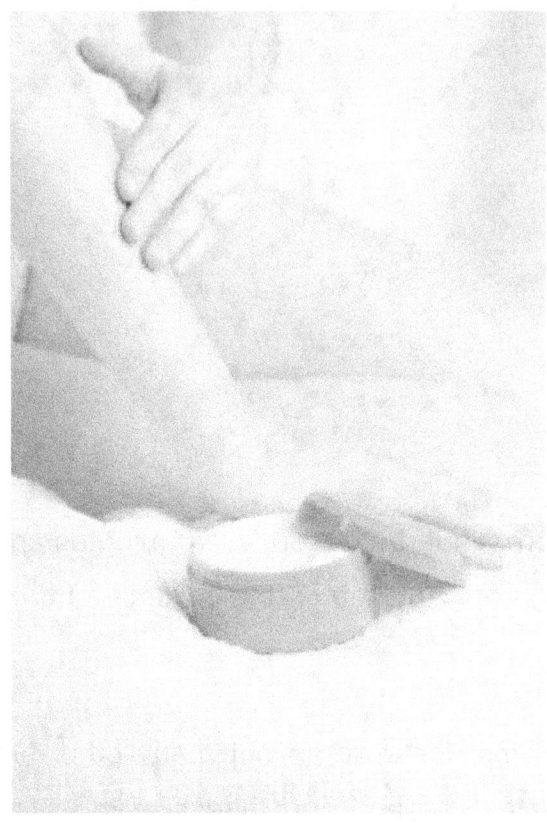

Acne & Pimples

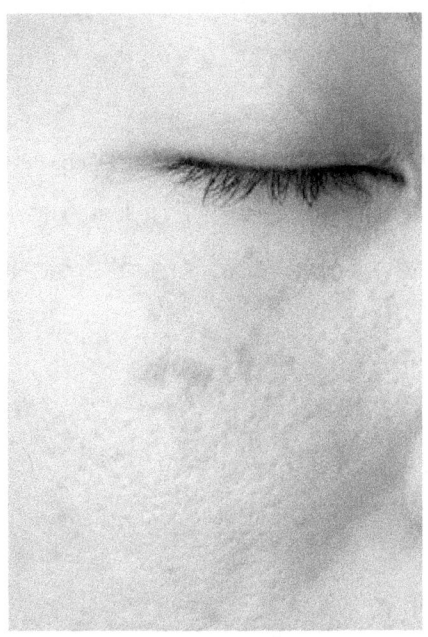

1. Eggy Idea

Eggs may stink, but they can work wonders for your skin conditions. It isn't just your hair that benefits from eggs, your skin can also attain a glow and smoothness that nothing else can give. Combine it with some other herbal cures, and you can easily get rid of the most stubborn acne.

Ingredients

1 egg white

1 tablespoon of honey

½ teaspoon of turmeric

1 teaspoon of cinnamon

Methods

Beat the egg white and then add all other ingredients to it. Mix them well and apply to the affected areas. Let it stay on for about 15-20 minutes and wash off with lukewarm water. Repeat this process once every day. You will get rid of the acne in 1-2 months, depending on how bad it is.

2. <u>Neem Oatmeal Scrub</u>

Neem is known for its antibacterial and antifungal properties. It is a great cure for many kinds of skin conditions, especially for acne. But keep in mind that neem is not suitable for everyone. There are some people who are allergic to it, so try it on a small spot before using it on your face.

Ingredients

2 tablespoons of neem leaves

¼ teaspoon of turmeric

2 tablespoons of ground oatmeal

½ teaspoon of tea tree oil

1 teaspoon of milk

Methods

Mix all of the ingredients together and then apply to face. Rub gently in upward motions and leave on for 10 minutes. Wash off with tap water and then with cold water. This will not only cure the acne, it will also help to even the skin tone and make your skin softer.

3. <u>Pimple Ridding Tea</u>

This tea will help cleanse your system internally, helping to remove the cause of pimples and acne. Try it for a while to see how it affects you. Do not continue drinking if you feel any side effects.

Ingredients

20 grams Herba Taraxaci

20 grams Fructus Aurantii Immaturus

20 grams Flos Lonicerae

Methods

Take about 1.5 liters of water in a pot and add all of the herbs to it. Boil and then reduce the heat. Let cook for 50 minutes and then use as tea for the whole day. You will have to consume the whole pot in one day.

4. Glowy, Wrinkle-Free Skin

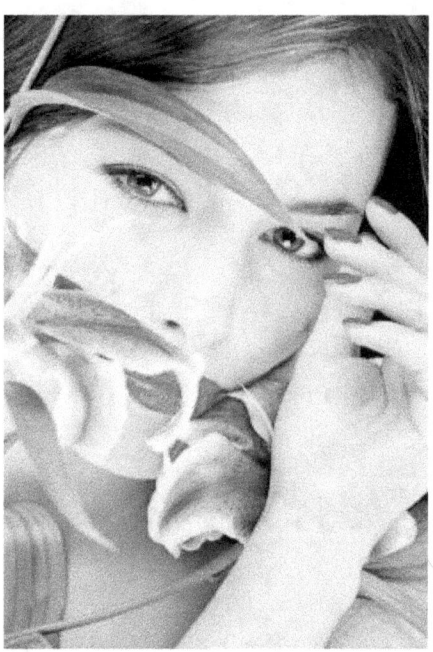

This tea can work for all those who feel that their skin is sagging, looking dull and getting too full of wrinkles. The complexion and elasticity of your skin will also improve.

Ingredients

30 grams Poria

60 grams Phizom Polygonati

60 grams Fructus Lycii

Methods

Take 3 liters of water and add all of the herbs to it. Bring to a boil, lower the heat and cook for another 60 minutes. You should cook it to the point where only 2 liters of tea is left. Strain, let cool and drink up. You can store this in the fridge and consume as much as you like.

5. Inner Skin Cleanser

As much as external skin care is important, it is also necessary that you pay attention to the inner functioning of the body. With the help of this tea you can make sure that a thorough internal cleansing takes place. This will keep your skin clean, clear and healthy. Note though that if you have a sensitive stomach you should avoid drinking too much of this tea.

Ingredients

50 grams Radiz Codonopsis Pilosulae

100 grams Phizoma Polygonati Odorati

Honey as per needed

Methods

Pour 3 liters of water in a pan and add the herbs to it. Do not add honey. Bring the liquid to a boil and then lower heat, simmering for another 60 minutes. When only 2 liters is left, strain and let cool. Add honey, if you like to make your tea sweet and consume as much as you like. Store in fridge and use as you like.

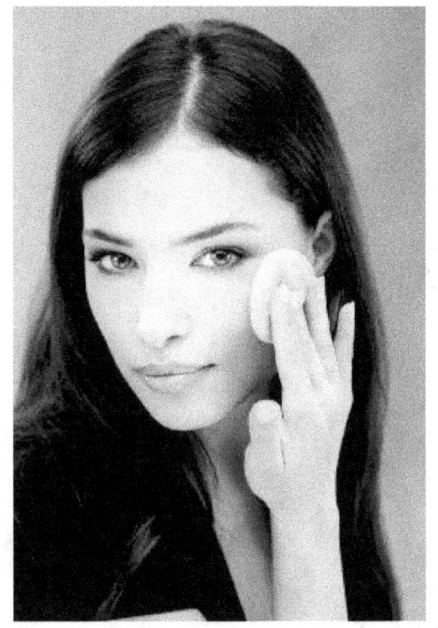

Lose the Pounds

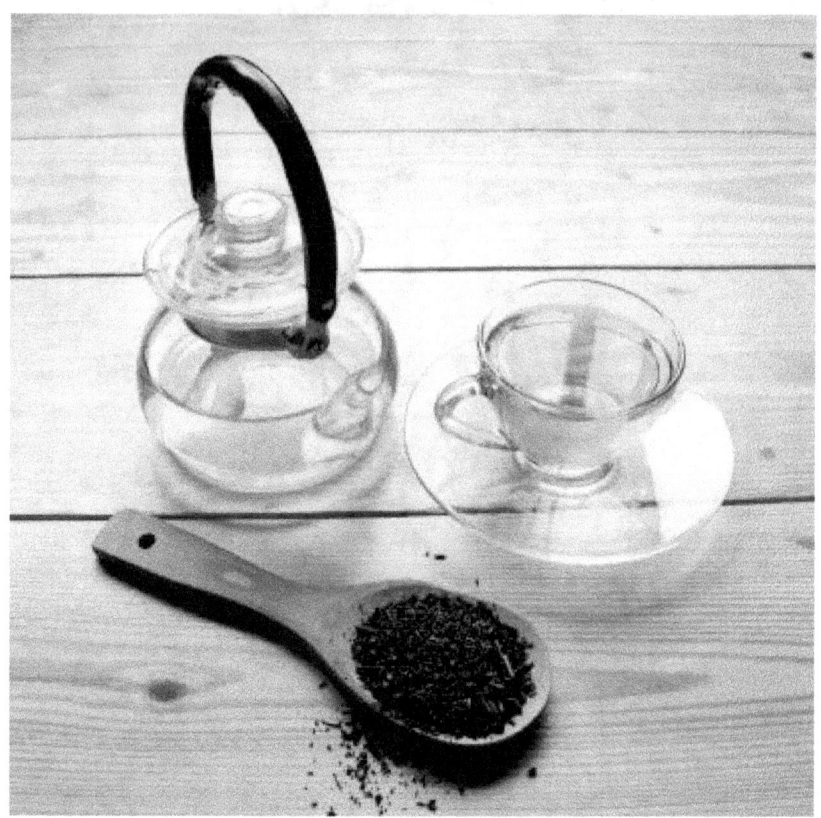

1. <u>Slimming Tea #1</u>

Becoming overweight is a concern for a vast majority of people these days. Instead of opting for the slim pills available in the market that have many side effects, try using these herbal remedies.

Ingredients

One part dandelion leaf

One part slippery elm bark

Two parts nettle leaf

One part senna leaf

One part marshmallow root

Two parts Eluthero root

Half part sweet cinnamon bark

One-fourth part fennel seeds

Half part orange peel

Half part ginger root

Methods

Mix all of the herbs together and add to water. Make tea, strain and consume throughout the day. The tea is mild so it will not affect your stomach. Don't try taking it on an empty stomach though. You will notice results within a month.

2. <u>Slimming Tea #2</u>

This tea is a three month on, 1 month rest kind of formula. You will have to take it for three months straight, leave a month off and then start again. Make sure you do not stop taking food. This tea will help you reduce weight and eliminate cellulite from your body. Keep a light hand on food intake though.

Ingredients

60 grams Fructus Crataegi

60 grams Folium Nelumbinis

Methods

Take 3 liters of water in a pot and add the herbs to it. Bring to a boil, lower the heat and simmer for another 60 minutes. When the tea is reduced to 1.3 liters, strain the herbs and let cool. This will yield 3 servings. Make sure you drink only one serving a day. You can refrigerate the rest for the next day.

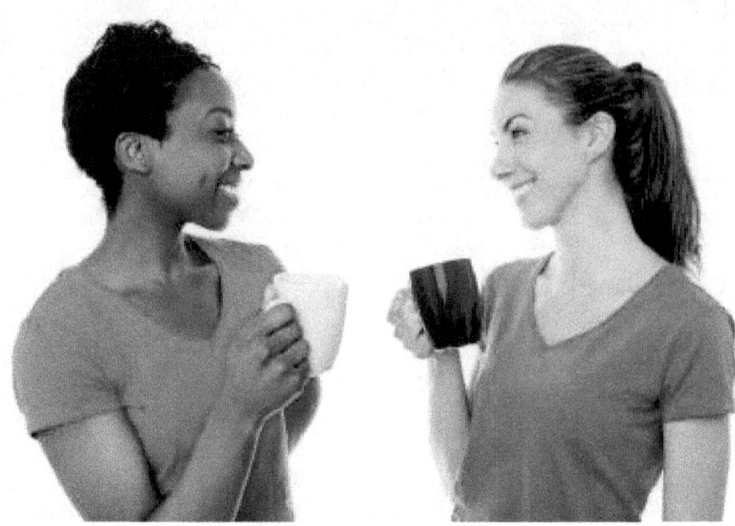

3. <u>Slimming Tea #3</u>

Here is another tea that will help you increase the metabolism and lose those pesky pounds.

Ingredients

3 tablespoons of grated ginger root (fresh)

2 pieces of dried garcinia fruit

½ a teaspoon of black seed

1 teaspoon of hawthorn berry

1 tablespoon of hibiscus

Some orange peel

Methods

Take 4 cups of cold water and pour in a pot. Add all the herbs and cover the lid. Bring to a boil, lower heat and let cook for 20 minutes. Strain the tea and serve hot or cold. You can also add a teaspoon of honey or stevia for sweet tea. ½ a lemon can also be added.

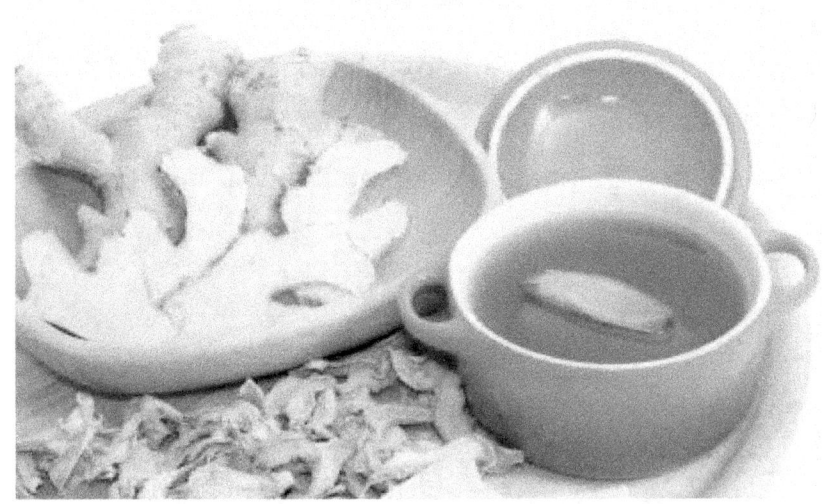

Conclusion

These are some of the most effective herbal healing recipes. Try them and see how they work for you. Just remember to try them on patches or in small amounts to find out whether they suit you or not. Do not use anything that you may be allergic to.

Best of luck!

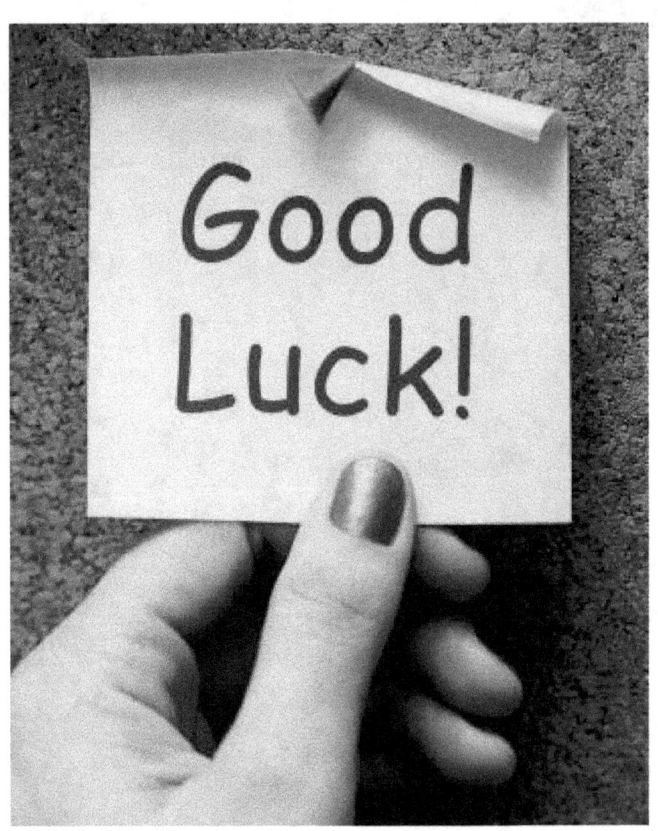